SLEEP

JOHNS HOPKINS
UNIVERSITY PRESS

AARHUS UNIVERSITY PRESS

CHRISTINE PARSONS

sleep

SLEEP

© Christine Parsons
and Johns Hopkins University Press 2023
Layout and cover: Camilla Jørgensen, Trefold
Cover photograph: Poul Ib Henriksen
Publishing editor: Karina Bell Ottosen
Translated from the Danish by Heidi Flegal
Printed by Narayana Press, Denmark
Printed in Denmark 2023

ISBN 978-1-4214-4608-0 (pbk)
ISBN 978-1-4214-4609-7 (ebook)

Library of Congress Control Number: 2022938146

*Special discounts are available for bulk purchases of this
book. For more information, please contact Special Sales at
specialsales@jh.edu.*

Published in the United States by:

Johns Hopkins University Press
2715 North Charles Street
Baltimore, MD 21218-4363
www.press.jhu.edu

Published with the generous support of the
Aarhus University Research Foundation

Purchase in Denmark: ISBN 978-87-7219-423-3

Aarhus University Press
Finlandsgade 29
8200 Aarhus N
Denmark
www.aarhusuniversitypress.dk

PEER
REVIEWED

MIX
Paper
FSC FSC® C010651

CONTENTS

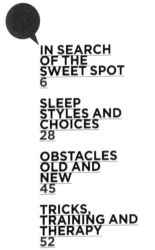

IN SEARCH OF THE SWEET SPOT

AN EXCELLENT SET OF LUNGS

"We were so worried. We had to keep checking that you were still breathing!" My parents love to recount how my arrival robbed them of sleep for almost an entire year. Their new baby had an excellent set of lungs, but seemed incapable of sleeping for more than two hours at a time. After months of short naps punctuated with crying, I finally slept for several hours. Rather than relief, they were beset with worry. What had brought about this drastic change? Would I ever wake again? Should they be on their way to the emergency room? Their extended sleep loss probably interfered with their ability to decipher this new, positive development. As many new parents will attest, those first few months with a newborn can wreak havoc on sleep patterns.

We become acutely aware of the impact of sleep in its absence. Who hasn't complained about tiredness, irritability or hunger after a less-than-adequate night's rest? While it is recommended that adults get between 7 and 9 hours' sleep, the likelihood that you fall within this range varies depending on the country you inhabit. In the United States, for example, the average sleep time falls at the lower end of the spectrum, with 35% of adults not getting the recommended minimum of 7 hours of sleep. In Sweden, adults do somewhat better, with only a small proportion (5%) of their population sleeping less than 6 hours.

These cross-country differences are reported even before adults join the workforce. A survey of almost 17,500 university students from 24 countries also reported very different average sleep times. Students in countries such as Thailand, Japan, Taiwan and Korea clustered around the 6.5-hour mark, while students in Spain and Romania reported getting about 8 hours.

Aside from differences across countries, about one fifth of university students get less than 7 hours' sleep per night. General population figures estimate that at least one third of adults report some sleep difficulty or other. Many of us are not getting enough sleep.

A large body of scientific studies now shows that too little sleep over time is linked to negative health consequences. These range from an increased risk of cardiovascular disease and stroke to diabetes and obesity, and early death. Even short-term sleep deprivation can have harmful effects, particularly reducing our capacity to pay attention.

Serious drops in attention, a hallmark of disrupted sleep, can be lethal. For driving performance, sleep deprivation can have effects equivalent to blood alcohol levels considered to be hazardous. Adults deprived of sleep for 17–19 hours in a lab experiment, and then tested on a driving simulator, performed at least as poorly as adults with a blood alcohol level of 0.05%, the legal limit in many countries. Thousands of car crashes every year can be traced back to a drowsy driver.

While many of us are aware of the consequences of too little sleep, there is growing evidence that we can also get too *much* sleep. Our best understanding is that there is a 'sweet spot' for what appears to be healthy sleep. Somewhere between 'not too little' and 'not too much' seems to be best for brain health and general functioning.

This sweet spot idea also applies to other areas of life, such as body weight, where 'too light' and 'too heavy' both entail health risks. In many cases, oversleeping is a side effect or an indicator of another health issue, like depression or a viral infection. What we do understand is that good-quality sleep, and a reasonable amount of it, is fundamental to well-being.

WHY DO WE SLEEP?

Across a life span of 80 years, we sleep for roughly 232,960 hours, or around 10,000 full days. We often consider sleep as wasted time. Yet our clear biological drive to sleep, and its occurrence across species, suggests that sleep provides benefits that outweigh its costs. And it is costly, depriving us of time we could otherwise spend interacting with others, foraging, learning. It renders us vulnerable to threats from the environment, unaware of our surroundings. Given the sacrifices we make to sleep, as the American sleep scientist Allan Rechtschaffen eloquently noted: "If sleep does not serve an absolutely vital function, then it is the biggest mistake the evolutionary process has ever made."

For years, scientists have tried to answer the question of why we sleep. Another American scientist Dr J Allan Hobson once joked that "The only known function of sleep is to cure sleepiness". Consider how we spend our time: two thirds awake, and one third asleep. We accomplish more than one function while awake, from eating and drinking to working or socialising. It seems reasonable to expect that we also accomplish more than one function while asleep. Indeed, many sleep functions have now been identified, ranging from restoring important peripheral tissues like skin and muscles, to clearing waste products in the brain built up over the day, to supporting memory and emotion processing. While it may not be the most satisfying of answers, it seems that sleep may serve *many* crucial functions.

One method for obtaining scientific evidence of sleep functions involves examining people when they are deprived of sleep, either deliberately or circumstantially. By observing the effects of going without sleep, we can get a sense of the purposes it serves, much like the process of removing parts of a bicycle and checking what still works.

There are numerous extreme cases of people voluntarily staying awake for unfathomable periods. Back in 1964, a seventeen-year-old student, Randy Gardner, undertook a project that would have lifelong consequences. Randy had moved to San Diego and decided he would need to pull out all the stops to win a science fair in the big city. With the help of two friends, he concocted a plan to attempt to break the world record for time awake. After 11 days, waves of severe nausea and memory loss, Randy got into the record books.

It was not easy. According to a scientist overseeing the experiment, each time Randy closed his eyes during the 11-day period, he immediately fell asleep. His friends had a hard fought battle to keep him awake, particularly during the night. Remarkably, at the end of his ordeal, he slept for just 14 hours and soon reported returning to what felt like 'normal'.

However, reflecting in a 2017 interview, Randy described being haunted by his teenage stunt, blaming it for his "unbearable" insomnia later in life. The *Guinness Book of World Records* has since removed the category of going without sleep because of the health risks involved.

Among the others who have attempted lengthy periods without sleep was Peter Tripp, the American radio DJ. He managed an 8-day stint in a glass booth in Times Square, New York City, in 1959. After about 105 hours, Tripp began to lose touch with reality, experiencing severe hallucinations. The psychiatrist overseeing Tripp noted "He was a sick man". After the stunt, Tripp's life took a series of downturns: he lost his job, was involved in serious financial scandals, and his wife divorced him.

However, as striking as these cases are, they are not our primary means to understand sleep deprivation and its consequences. Anyone willing to undertake such an extended ordeal may not represent 'the average person', and the data obtained does not tell us much about everyday sleep processes.

Instead, a lot of what we know about sleep comes from tightly controlled lab-based studies where volunteers are kept awake for shorter periods. Typically these studies restrict sleep for 24 to 48 hours, or ask people to sleep a bit less than they otherwise would. Even these short periods of disruption can have measurable, typically negative effects on the body, behaviour and brain.

Take our immune system, where even brief sleep deprivation can have an impact, for instance on how adults respond to a vaccine. For vaccines to work the body needs to produce specific proteins, antibodies, in response to the invading bacteria or virus. When people are partially deprived of sleep, perhaps having their sleep time halved for a few nights, then vaccinated, their bodies produce less of these critical antibodies. Ultimately, this can impact a vaccine's effectiveness.

A similar detrimental pattern is observed outside of the lab. People who get less than 6 hours of sleep per night are less likely to have an adequate antibody response, for instance to a hepatitis B vaccine, than longer sleepers. On the flip side, if you get more than 7 hours of sleep you tend to be more resistant to catching a cold when exposed to the virus in the lab. Sleep duration is not the only important variable here, either. Poor sleep efficiency – spending time in bed but not sleeping – may also lowers resistance to the common cold virus.

Think back on your last poor night's sleep. How

was your mood the next day? Your ability to cope under pressure? This, too, seems to be intricately tied to how you sleep. Numerous lab experiments have restricted people's opportunity to sleep, checking that volunteers are still awake by monitoring their brain activity, or asking them to fill in questionnaires at frequent intervals. After ensuring a sleep-restricted night, researchers are then free to probe emotional responses using standard psychological tests.

One elegant example of such a study took a group of teenagers and tinkered with their sleep opportunity over three weeks. For five nights, the teens were allowed to sleep their regular, and age-appropriate, 10 hours. For another five nights, they were only allowed 6.5 hours. With just a few hours less over five nights, the teenagers themselves noted feeling more tense, angry, confused and frustrated.

The sleep deprivation effects were also clear to the teenagers' parents, who noted greater irritability and poorer emotion regulation in their children. What makes these findings especially important is that the teenagers were restricting their sleep over a short period, and not by a huge quantity. It seems that even partial, never mind total, sleep deprivation can affect mood regulation.

Similar negative patterns have also been found in adults. When studying healthy adults, researchers are allowed to ramp up the conditions of sleep deprivation compared to what is ethically acceptable for teenage volunteers. One American study from 2005 allowed adults to sleep for only 4 hours, half the normal, recommended nightly amount, over a longer period of 12 days. As the experiment rolled on, the adults on the 4-hour sleep regimen became progressively less optimistic about the future and less social. They also reported more bodily discomfort, such as pain and an upset stomach, peaking at day 6, at about the halfway point of the study.

Some good news, however: After a single 12-hour recovery period in bed, participants reported feeling back to their initial baseline levels, including for self-reported optimism and pain. Although this return to baseline coincided with the experiment ending – which may indicate participants' relief that their ordeal was over – the scientists suggested that quick recovery from sleep deprivation may indeed be possible.

FOOD AS A CONSOLATION PRIZE

If you tend to reach for sugary, high-fat foods like a Danish pastry or pizza after a sleepless night, you are not alone. People who habitually sleep less than 6 hours a night are more likely to end up with an unhealthy body mass index. One reason is that we seem to compensate for sleep loss by increasing our calorie intake.

Nestled within the sprawling Ivy League campus of the University of Pennsylvania in Philadelphia is a laboratory dedicated to studying sleep as rigorously as possible. The lab is custom-built so that the lighting can be precisely controlled, along with the ambient temperature and noise levels. It is stocked with a range of physiological monitoring equipment, along with more mundane items like a selection of board games, books, a TV and even a kitchen. These all become very necessary if you are going to keep participants in the lab, without breaks, for a full week.

The experiment began in 2010 and took several years to complete. During this time, 44 volunteers came to the lab and were monitored by the research team at regular intervals. They were asked not to do any exercise, and wore wrist-monitors that allowed researchers to keep an eye on their compliance. Their sleep hours were also measured and, after a few 'baseline' days, restricted to 4 hours for five consecutive nights. Confined to the lab for the full week, participants were allowed to order any food item they wanted from a menu. Every meal and every snack was weighed and recorded by the research team.

When the volunteers were sleep-restricted, they responded by bumping up their daily calorie intake significantly average, compared to after their fully-rested nights. Rather than simply a general upping of food intake, the extra calories came mainly from late-night desserts and salty snacks. Men particularly ate additional food at night compared to women, even though earlier in the day, their intake was about the same.

Sleeping only 4 hours over multiple nights is unpleasant, but even shorter periods of deprivation can lead to a large increase in food intake. A 2008 experiment gradually reduced women's sleep over four nights, from a healthy 8 hours, to 7 hours, then 6 for two nights, then to just 4 hours for one night. At the end of this narrowing sleep window, women had increased their calorie intake by about 20%. This also resulted in a change in weight patterns: On average, the women had gained almost half a kilogram at the end of the four days. We can conclude that even gradual reductions in sleep time can make it harder to calibrate our calorie intake to our metabolic needs, and to maintain a healthy body weight.

MEMORY AID

There is now considerable scientific evidence that sleep enhances memory. This applies to different types of memory, like the kind we use to recall stories or to perform skills such as riding a bike or playing the piano. When trying to learn a new skill, we need to practise repeatedly, or 'train', and then to 'consolidate' that learning. We may practise riding a bike, for instance, but it takes a while to see the full benefit of that practice. This period of consolidation, after the practice itself ends, goes on for some time, depending on the skill in question.

If adults are deprived of sleep after training, when consolidation has to happen, they can have considerable difficulty acquiring that new skill. And there seems to be a critical window in which sleep has to happen. Looking at one type of skill learning, a rather boring task of telling two pictures apart, one study reported that sleep had to occur within 30 hours of training for participants to improve their performance.

While we typically think of sleep in 8-hour blocks, when it comes to skill-learning, even a nap can be helpful. In fact, a nap can provide similar benefits to a full night's sleep for certain tasks. Again, using the picture-discrimination task, one experiment trained adults in the morning, and then allowed some of the volunteers to take an afternoon nap of 60 or 90 minutes.

Other less fortunate adults were told to go about their day as normal, with no nap. When everyone was tested again at 7 p.m. that evening, the nappers were already better at the task than the 'no-nap' group. Nap length was not crucial either; 60 and 90 minutes of napping produced similar results, as long as the napper reached the deeper stages of sleep.

Additional lines of research emphasising the importance of sleep for memory have looked at one devastating disease: Alzheimer's. Sleep problems are frequent among people with the disease, who tend to nod off during the day and wake repeatedly during the night. In fact, sleep disruption is so common in patients with Alzheimer's that scientists now are examining whether broken sleep patterns, like difficulties staying awake or waking up too often, could be an early sign of the disease.

The link between Alzheimer's and sleep might run in both directions. That is, Alzheimer's itself might disrupt sleep patterns, while poor sleep may also increase an individual's risk of developing Alzheimer's. A 2017 analysis of 27 studies conducted around the world, including nearly 70,000 participants, estimated that as many as 15% of Alzheimer's cases could be attributed to sleep problems, although the reasons for this link are not entirely clear.

A hallmark of Alzheimer's disease is the presence of clumps of beta-amyloid, a waste product of metabolism. Sleep may be critical to clearing out beta-amyloid, and other metabolic debris that builds up over the course of the day. That is, sleep functions like a 'plumbing system' for the brain and prevents the problematic build-up of beta-amyloid. Laboratory studies with mice suggest that this might be the case: when mice are chronically deprived of sleep, beta-amyloid plaques accumulate more rapidly in their brains. The negative effects of poor sleep on beta-amyloid levels are also under investigation in humans, with scientists increasingly focusing on this link. One landmark study in 2017 suggested that just one night of sleep deprivation affected beta-amyloid clearance in the human brain.

In this study, 17 healthy American adults were asked to sleep at the National Institutes of Health in Maryland, while their brain waves were measured. On one night, the volunteers had a night of their sleep disrupted, with a series of loud beeps played each time they sank into deep sleep. The next morning, the sleep-disrupted volunteers had the levels of beta-amyloid in the fluid around their brains and spinal cords measured. On another night, the participants again slept in the lab in an identical set-up, but without the sleep-disrupting tones. The results were striking: The more deep sleep disruption participants experienced, the greater the levels of beta amyloid the researchers measured.

With these findings in mind, it is easy to imagine how

chronic sleep deprivation, if untreated over several years, could increase the accumulation of beta-amyloid, and therefore the risk and progression of Alzheimer's.

NO SKIMPING

Early in his campaign for the US presidential election in 2016, the Republican candidate Donald Trump made several public statements about his sleep style: "I have a great temperament for success. ... You know, I'm not a big sleeper. I like three hours, four hours, I toss, I turn, I beep-de-beep, I want to find out what's going on."

Trump's irregular and shortened sleep times often have him on Twitter, frequently posting commentary at 5 or 6 a.m. Notable examples include his tweet "Despite the negative press covfefe", a partial sentence sent just after midnight in May 2017, and accusations of voter fraud in Iowa in 2016, sent at 1:38 a.m.

While there is evidence that some individuals do need less sleep than others, for most the negative effects of skimping on sleep accumulate over time. Of even greater concern is the fact that we are often unaware of increasing cognitive deficits with continued short sleep. One 2003 study assigned adults to sleep 4, 6 or 8 hours a night over two weeks, monitoring their performance on tests measuring attention, working memory and mental arithmetic. The adults getting 4 and 6 hours did progressively worse as the days passed. Contrary to what we often imagine, the volunteers showed no signs of 'adapting' to sleep deprivation.

The researchers also asked the volunteers about how sleepy they felt. Initially, they reported high levels of sleepiness. But by the end of the two weeks of sleep restriction, when cognitive performance was at its worst, they reported feeling only slightly sleepy. This finding may help us to understand why people often continue with a short sleep pattern: They believe they have adapted to less sleep because they do not feel particularly sleepy.

Another US president, Bill Clinton, also reported being on the short end of the sleep spectrum, getting 5 to 6 hours a night during his eight years in the White House in the 1990s. Appearing in a 2007 interview with Jon Stewart on *The Daily Show*, he stated that many of his mistakes as a politician stemmed from tiredness. "I do believe sleep deprivation has a lot to do with some of the edginess of Washington today," he said, suggesting that "America would work better" if its leaders got more sleep.

THE PERILS OF DRIVER FATIGUE

Car accidents provide devastating, concrete evidence of just how harmful sleep deprivation can be. It is estimated that 7% of all crashes in the US involve driver drowsiness. For fatal crashes, some 16% are thought to have involved a drowsy driver. A 2018 large-scale American study of more than 6,000 drivers involved in car accidents examined driver sleep in the 24 hours preceding the accident. By splitting the drivers into those who had caused the crash they were involved in and those who had not, the American researcher Brian Tefft could look at the critical role of sleep. The results were not surprising in light of our general understanding of driver fatigue.

Drivers who reported sleeping less than 7 hours were more likely to cause an accident than those who said they slept for 7 to 9 hours. Anything less than 7 hours was associated with an increased risk of causing an accident. Drivers in the most risky, 'less than 4 hours of sleep' category were disproportionately involved in single-vehicle accidents – which are about three times more likely to cause a fatality than multiple-vehicle accidents.

Tefft noted that drivers who had experienced recent changes in their sleep or work schedules also had an increased risk of causing an accident. Unsurprisingly, drivers who reported typically feeling drowsy on awakening, an indicator of unrefreshing or insufficient sleep, also had an increased risk. While these findings – that schedule changes or poor-quality sleep patterns heighten driving-related risks – are worrying, they do provide good reason to educate drivers, healthcare providers and policy-makers on the importance of sleep for driver safety.

THE CIRCADIAN RHYTHM

According to British government documents dating back as far as 1519, King Henry VII once told an adviser he wished to "slepe and drem apon the matter, and geff me an answer apon the morning." 'Sleep on it' has long been the popular advice given to those with a dilemma to solve.

One of the most cited examples of sleep as an aid to problem-solving comes from the nineteenth-century

German chemist Friedrich Kekulé. He was a key figure in early modern organic chemistry, studying carbon-based compounds – the building blocks of life.

In a speech given at a scientific meeting in 1890, Kekulé recalled the details of a dream he had 30 years prior, while dozing in front of a fire in the Belgian city of Ghent. In this dream he saw atoms dance around, form into strings, and move about, snake-like. He then saw a serpent take shape, and swallow its own tail. This image led him to the idea of the cyclic structure of the carbon-based compound benzene. Whether this dream sequence really occurred or was merely a tall tale told to amuse fellow scientists, it has become a favourite anecdote among psychologists, philosophers and historians of science about the power of sleep.

Otto Loewi, a German-born pharmacologist is perhaps better known for the method with which he came up with his experiment than for the discovery that earned him the Nobel Prize in Physiology or Medicine in 1936. In describing his experiment, he told how he dreamed the procedure that would show that the transmission of nerve impulses was chemical, rather than electrical. He woke up one night to write his dream down, but alas! The next morning he found his own handwriting illegible. Fortunately, his dream reoccurred the next night and this time he woke and immediately went to the laboratory to perform his 'dream' experiment. Loewi's work also led to the discovery of acetylcholine, the first brain chemical ever identified – which is now understood to generate states of wakefulness.

There are two major, inter-related drivers of whether we want to be asleep or be awake. The first is a signal from a structure deep inside the brain, a biological pacemaker called the *suprachiasmatic nucleus*, SCN for short, which controls the day-and-night rhythm that regulates our feeling awake or tired. The second driver is a chemical signal from the compound adenosine, which accumulates in the brain during periods of wakefulness. The longer you are awake, the more adenosine builds up, creating 'sleep pressure', an urge to sleep. The balance between these two drivers, the SCN-based pacemaker and adenosine levels, impacts our daytime wakefulness and our night-time sleepiness.

Most living creatures – plants, humans and other animals – have biological clocks that help to adapt physiology to fluctuations over the day. This regular adaptation, termed the '*circadian* rhythm', derives from the Latin words *circa*, 'around', and *dies*, 'day'.

As a nod to the importance of circadian rhythms, the 2017 Nobel Prize in Medicine or Physiology was awarded to a trio of American researchers for their discoveries on the molecules that control them. The circadian clock is not only reactive to changes in the day; it also anticipates them, and alters our physiology accordingly. Our circadian rhythm affects not only our sleep, but also how we eat, and our blood pressure and body temperature.

The SCN is the central controller of our circadian

rhythm, but despite its far-reaching role, it is actually tiny. It contains around 20,000 brain cells, a mere pinch out of the estimated 100 billion or so cells in a human brain. To track time, the SCN uses daylight, the most reliably re-occurring signal in our environment.

Light travels to the SCN from the optic nerve in our eyes. The SCN uses this light signal to keep us to a 24-hour rhythm. Regular exposure to both light and darkness is the primary way we stay synchronised to the solar day. While light is one means to manipulate our circadian rhythm, we can also manipulate the second driver, sleep pressure, via another remarkably common means.

AND SO WE TURN TO STIMULANTS

It is Tuesday morning. As usual, my day begins at the office coffee machine. I'm normally in luck, like today. Someone else was here before me, and the machine is warmed up, ready to sputter into action. The boiler heats. The beans grind. The hot water whistles and gurgles. A cacophony of sound as brown liquid accumulates in my mug. The aroma of coffee percolates to my colleagues nearby. It won't be long before one of them is drawn to the machine.

Coffee is so popular we often think of it as a drink, rather than a medium for delivering a psychoactive drug: caffeine. In fact, caffeine is the most widely-used stimulant in the world, present in chocolate, coffee, tea and energy drinks. Its effects can be enormously positive: elevating mood, promoting vigilance, reducing sleepiness. When we are sleep-deprived, a good dose of caffeine can be as effective as prescription-only stimulants like amphetamine and modafinil for restoring alertness and motor performance.

Caffeine takes aim at our chemical sleep driver, adenosine, which acts as a chemical egg-timer for how long we've been awake. As time passes, adenosine levels build, tracking our awake time. Caffeine can temporarily mute the effects of adenosine by attaching to the brain-receptor sites where adenosine normally binds. Adenosine levels therefore do not send the same 'sleepiness' signal when caffeine is present, creating a temporary sense of alertness.

The relationship between caffeine and sleep is especially interesting to me as a Scandinavian resident, where caffeine consumption is among the highest in the world. In my adopted country, Danes consume an average of roughly 8.7 kg of coffee per capita per year. And it's a common habit: 80% of the population aged 15–75 say they are regular coffee drinkers.

Coffee did not arrive in Europe until the seventeenth century, but legend has it that it was discovered growing wild in Ethiopia in the ninth century: Kaldi, a solitary goatherd, noticed that his animals became very lively after eating berries from a certain tree. He shared his discovery with the abbot of the local monastery, who boiled a drink with dried berries from the tree. The abbot and his monks used this drink to stay awake throughout the long hours required to properly observe their night-time prayers.

While its stimulant effects can be beneficial if you

need to stay awake, caffeine clearly disrupts sleep. It typically makes it harder to fall asleep quickly, reduces total sleep time and worsens perceived sleep quality. While the amount of caffeine in the bloodstream peaks around 30 minutes after drinking a cup of coffee, the important property for sleep is the length of time it stays in your system. On average, it takes 5 to 7 hours to clear half of your coffee's caffeine from your body. However, caffeine-clearing capacity varies immensely, depending on a person's body weight, gender, kidney function and so on. Indeed, as we age, our ability to remove caffeine from our bodies declines, making us more sensitive to sleep disruption with caffeine intake.

They may be less pleasant than a cup of coffee, but caffeine pills provide distinct advantages for assessing the effects of the drug on sleep. For researchers, it is easier to control the exact dose, and also to remove the effect of volunteer expectations – by not telling study subjects whether their pill contains caffeine or not (that is, by using a 'placebo' pill). Caffeine pills are not sold here in Denmark, but they are widely used in other European countries. In Germany, a survey of students found that about 10.5% had taken caffeine pills at some point to enhance their academic performance.

Cognitive boosts aside, caffeine pills are regularly used in research studies to examine the importance of timing and dosing for sleep. One week-long American study, published in 2013, gave volunteers either caffeine pills or non-caffeinated 'placebo' pills to take on different days, and at different intervals before bed: right before, within 3 hours, or 6 hours before. Even when taking caffeine pills 6 hours before bed, volunteers slept around an hour less in total than when taking a placebo pill.

The study participants reported noticing disturbed sleep when taking their pill either 3 hours before bed, or right before, but there was no statistically significant difference between their sleep time reports for the 6-hour interval. The extent of the caffeine-related sleep disturbance was obvious from the measures of actual sleep braining activity. The volunteers' sleep diaries showed a different picture: people were not aware of caffeine's negative impact.

According to the scientists, when volunteers took caffeine 6 hours before bed, they likely experienced short awakenings, which are pretty tricky to recall. How does this translate into the real world? If caffeine is taken in the early afternoon, as in the 6-hour condition, it may affect sleep more subtly – less noticeably. If the effects are hard to perceive, it is easy to see why many of us drink coffee well beyond our morning routines.

Awareness of the effects of caffeine is widespread, and its benefits and harms for health are frequently debated. Possibly as a result of this uncertainty, market-sales figures, mainly from the US, indicate a marked shift to decaffeinated coffee.

However, there are currently no labelling restrictions for 'decaffeinated' products. An analysis of various Starbucks decaf offerings, for instance, showed wide variation in actual caffeine content, at 0–14 mg per serving. Even within the same café, there was between 3 and 16 mg of caffeine in a 'decaf' shot. Such quantities may not be as detrimental to sleep as a triple-shot latte or a 400-mg caffeine pill, but some sensitive individuals might still feel an effect. But in general, three to four cups of brewed coffee a day, about 300–400 mg of caffeine, is deemed safe for most healthy adults.

SLEEP STYLES AND CHOICES

SOCIAL JETLAG

About 80% of volunteers in a large European study reported using an alarm to wake up on work days. Needing an alarm is a good indicator that there is a gap between your natural wake time and that imposed by societal demands. Referred to as "social jetlag", it is a gap experienced by many. Like travel jetlag, social jetlag is associated with a host of negative symptoms such as drowsiness, poorer task performance and worsened mood.

However, a major difference between travel and social jetlag is how often the two are experienced. Travel jetlag tends to be an infrequent, unfortunate result of holiday travel. Social jetlag, on the other hand, occurs as part of our normal daily lives, and can continue for years when sleep-skewing schedules don't align with natural wake times. Over the long term, social jetlag can be associated with health conditions like diabetes and cardiovascular disease.

Some people are impacted more by social jetlag than others. For 'night owls', the discrepancy between a preferred late-starter rhythm and typical early-morning work or school start times is greater. For 'morning larks', early start times may be more in sync with natural awakenings, and will not be an issue. Larks reach peak alertness soon after waking, and they are best able to do cognitive tasks early in the day. Not so for owls, who are most alert and active in the evening.

Besides preferring to stay up late, or rise early, night owls and morning larks often differ in personality, too. Morning larks are, on average, slightly more conscientious, more co-operative and more persistent with their goals. Night owls tend to be more extroverted, less risk-averse and more impulsive.

The idea that having a night-time chronotype might be linked to a specific set of personality traits was the focus of a 2014 Ig Nobel Prize-winning study. The Ig Nobel prize is a Harvard-based award to celebrate imaginative research projects that "first make people laugh, then make them think". While night owls may not find this characterization so amusing, the British and Australian researchers linked being a night owl with the higher Dark Triad traits: narcissism, psychopathy and Machiavellianism. In their study of 263 men and women, those who habitually stayed up late reported more of the "dark" traits studied, than people who habitually rise early in the morning.

Perhaps not the most flattering portrayal – but other research suggests that night owls are also more creative and more intelligent. Although favourable and less favourable personality traits are associated with each chronotype, most of us – about 60% – fall between these extremes.

Chronotype also changes across the lifespan, with several clear shifts in preferred waking times. Children start off as early risers, then gradually move towards later awakenings. By around 17 or 18 years, American teenagers report average weekend bedtimes of 00:45. Their 'lateness' peaks somewhere around age 20, after which they start to shift back to earlier rising times. Preferring to stay up late or rise early is at least partly dictated by genetics, and the overall trends are reasonably constant across the lifespan. That is, if you are a real morning lark, you will tend to get up before your peers across your lifespan.

SLEEPING THE DAY AWAY

It's a familiar scenario for many parents. My colleague vents her frustration over a morning coffee break: "He's up half the night on that iPad, or iPhone, or i-something. Of course he can't get up in the morning. He's hardly slept!" She is the concerned mother of a teenage zombie, and she is growing tired of the struggle each morning to get him out of bed.

Teenagers are one of the most maligned groups when it comes to sleep and sleep patterns. Their propensity to stay up late and sleep in is a common source of parental aggravation. We know that late-night patterns are common for teenagers around the world, at least where studies have been carried out. Bedtimes become later and later with each passing year of adolescence, but adolescents have a longer estimated sleep need than adults, at around 8–10 hours.

When it comes to social jetlag, teenagers may be especially hard hit. Comparing sleep on weekdays and weekends, teenagers in many countries delay their weekend wake times by more than 2.5 hours, as compared to weekdays. This suggests a mismatch between teenagers' natural rhythms and current school start times.

If being a night owl is so universal for teenagers, why does school start so early? In the US, more than 90% of schools start classes before 8:30, with the average being 8:03. Getting to school can mean a very early start. In Denmark, similarly, schools generally start around 8 o'clock. Coming from Ireland, I am used to a gentler start time of 9:00. Irish school guidelines specify that schools should be open by 9:30 at the latest, with formal classes kicking into action by 9:50.

There have been important policy discussions on the issue of school start times. For example, the American Academy for Sleep Medicine issued a position statement in 2017 arguing that for teenagers, school should not start before 8:30. This recommendation has been supported by other major groups of scientists and health experts, including the American Academy of Pediatrics and the Centers for Disease Control and Prevention. Such a shift in start times would give teenagers more opportunity to get enough sleep during the week.

Some researchers in the UK have even called for school start times to shift to 10:00 for 16-year-olds, and 11:00 for 18-year-olds. But change is not easy. Some schools would have to re-arrange bus schedules, sports events and after-school activities. In fact, one large trial in the UK to test delayed school times was abandoned because too few schools signed up to take part. The researchers began recruitment in 2015, contacting thousands of schools and offering financial compensation, but found only two schools willing to participate.

Published in 2012, Norway tested a compromise, starting Monday mornings at 9:30, then sticking with 8:30 for the rest of the week. The researchers compared the late-Monday start group with a school that kept to their normal 8:30 start time. The later schedule was in place for two years, giving teachers an extra hour for a Monday-morning staff meeting. And the impact on the teenagers' sleep schedules? Those allowed to start an hour later on Mondays got an extra hour of sleep Sunday night, compared to their 'school as normal' peers. The 'intervention' group also showed slightly better reaction times when tested for alertness on their late-start Mondays, as compared to normal-start Fridays.

Besides extra costs, opponents of delaying school start times have raised other concerns. For example, will teens just stay up later if they can sleep a bit longer in the mornings? The Norwegian trial results suggest that this is not necessarily the case. Those in the late-start group actually did get an extra hour of sleep. Another study published in 2016 from an all-girls school in Singapore tested out the impact of delaying school start times by 45 minutes, pushing their start from 7:30 to 8:15. Students spent an extra 23 minutes in bed, an increase that was almost the same when measured again nine months later.

Another opposition point is a pragmatic one: Teenagers need to get used to early starts as training for the 'real world'. Parents often oppose school start times shifting for this reason, but there is good evidence that teenagers will naturally move back to better morning functioning as they get older. Adolescent night-owl behaviour is a phase, and by young and middle adulthood, circadian rhythms do shift to earlier bedtimes and awakenings. For elderly adults, in fact, this shift continues, leading to earlier and earlier bedtimes.

SOCIAL SLEEP

Millions of adults sleep next to a significant other – sharing a bed is a common practice globally. Throughout history, sleep patterns have been shaped by those around us, be it a partner or a larger group. However, research has tended to focus on the individual, largely ignoring the social context of sleep. Most sleep laboratories are built with one person in mind, which is a simpler technical set-up than wiring up two adults simultaneously.

Notwithstanding the focus on the individual, most scientists will acknowledge that couples' sleep patterns are tightly intertwined. If one has sleep difficulties, both are impacted. If one has extreme 'lark' or 'owl' tendencies, the other may find themselves woken at atypical times. Natural movement by one partner during the night can result in 'micro-awakenings' in the other. For many couples, however, the security and comfort of their partner's presence overrides such disturbances. Others find solutions such as separate beds or separate rooms helpful. Numerous well-known couples – the film director Baz Luhrmann and the Oscar-winning designer Catherine Martin, for example – celebrate separate bedrooms as 'marriage savers'.

It is probably a good idea to find a sleeping pattern that reduces couple conflict, for the sake of both day-time and night-time functioning. An American study from 2011 titled "Don't go to bed angry" found that when couples reported more conflict during the day, they also had worse sleep that night. Bad sleep sets up the conditions for conflict, and conflict makes for bad sleep. With an equally apt title – "Do sleepless nights mean worse fights?" – another group of researchers found that after poor sleep, couples were less able to resolve a conflict situation. This was true even when just one partner had a bad previous night's sleep.

SLEEP IN ATHLETES

"Well, I had real trouble sleeping that night." I was pestering my husband about how it felt to finish his first Ironman triathlon, a one-day endurance event that spans 140.6 miles. With his typical Danish reservedness, he did not have much to say. But his sleep, or lack of it, had stuck with him. When what we want most of all is to sleep – when we are so tired we can barely swim, bike or run another inch – it can elude us. For athletes, professional and amateur, sleep is considered a key factor in recovering after virtually any major sporting effort.

When asked about the most important component of his training, sprinter Usain Bolt responded: "Sleep." Bolt, who reportedly sleeps 8–10 hours a night, also regularly took naps right before his most spectacular performances, like his gold-medal wins in Beijing 2008. Similarly, LeBron James, one of the greatest basketball players of all time, claims he averages 12 hours of sleep a day, broken into 8–9 hours at night with extra daytime naps.

While some exceptional athletes have equally exceptional sleep routines, emulating their emphasis on sleep might be beneficial to the less talented amongst us. Scientists from Stanford University set out to look at what happens when sleep is encouraged in college-level athletes – instead of the typical set up of depriving the athletes of sleep and measuring performance drops, the California-based scientist Cheri Mah and her team did the opposite. Mah asked basketball players to get *more* sleep during the National Collegiate Athletic Association season and measured their resulting performance.

Eleven male players wore motion-sensing watches to estimate their sleep time, which came to about 6.68 hours a night on average. The players themselves thought they were getting much more sleep, about 7.8 hours according to their self-recorded sleep diaries. For two weeks they slept as usual, and their performance was measured on sprint drills, free throws and three-point shooting. Then they were asked to sleep as much as possible for five to seven weeks, aiming for 10 hours each night.

During the sleep-extension period, the players said they slept around 10.4 hours, while their watches said 8.45 on average. By either measure, they were getting more sleep. And the performance improvements were clear cut. Their sprint times got faster, dropping from 16.2 seconds to 15.5, and their free-throw accuracy rose by 9%. Unsurprisingly, their levels of daytime sleepiness also decreased, and their mood improved. Of course, a study of 11 players is a small one and improvements may also be due to the season progressing, but this level of performance enhancement is of a size that makes team managers and coaches pay attention.

A wide variety of elite sports teams and projects now place a special emphasis on their athletes' sleep. This trend has runners getting 10–12 hours of sleep per night, American football teams hiring consultants for advice on player sleep, and touring cyclists dozing on personal mattresses and pillows to ensure they get good-quality sleep.

CORPORATE NAPS

Sleep was once considered a leveller of men. The English poet Sir Philip Sidney, writing in the 1500s, referred to sleep as "the poor man's wealth, the prisoner's release, the indifferent judge between the high and low".

Later, however, in a 1719 sermon entitled "Vigilius, or, The Awakener", Cotton Mather, the famed American religious leader, called an excess of sleep "sinful", deriding those who sleep when they should be working. Sleep was regarded as an indulgence, a weakness best avoided. As founding father Benjamin Franklin, a prolific writer and renowned early riser, quipped in *Poor Richard's Almanack*: "there'll be sleeping enough in the grave".

Echoing these sentiments, some companies have glorified sleep deprivation and what can be achieved if you forgo sleep. Facebook have turned all-night coding sessions into events, 'hackathons', which are a celebrated part of their culture. One intern described a hackathon: "like a sleepover but for nerds … Except without the sleep." Elon Musk famously tweeted in November 2018 that "nobody ever changed the world on 40 hours a week". During a CBS interview he said, "Yeah, I'm sleeping on the factory floor, not because I think that's a fun place to sleep. You know. Terrible." Musk presents his sleep deprivation, his willingness to endure hardships, as necessary to his success. But is this truly the way to optimal workplace performance?

In the early hours of 21 August 2017, ten sailors aboard the *USS John S. McCain* were killed when their ship collided with an oil tanker in Singapore territorial waters. This came only a few months after the *USS Fitzgerald* and a container ship collided in Japanese waters in June 2017, killing seven sailors. Both ships were guided-missile destroyers.

The harrowing investigations that followed highlighted missed warnings, chains of error and desperate sailors attempting to save their fellow shipmates. The US Navy determined that fatigue and poor sleep management contributed to both fatal collisions. It has since changed its policy to allow all sailors working on aircraft carriers to get eight hours of uninterrupted sleep. The military's shifting stance on sleep is significant, as sleep deprivation among its personnel has, for decades, been viewed as unavoidable.

Poor sleep can also cost workplaces money. A 2011 report from Harvard Medical School, which telephone-surveyed over 7,000 workers, estimated that sleep difficulties were costing 2,280 US dollars in lost productivity for the average worker every year. When projected to a national scale, this estimate came to 63.2 billion dollars.

The analysis made one point clear: Workers were not missing work due to poor sleep. Rather, they attended work, but achieved less because of their fatigue levels. RAND corporation, a well-reputed, independent American research organisation, estimated that high-income countries lose up to 3% of their gross domestic product due to lack of sleep. Their research further suggested that more sleep could add billions of dollars in productivity to a nation's economy.

These findings on the effects of sleep issues on productivity have started to trickle into the policies of some workplaces. According to a Google spokesman, Jordan Newman, the company's offices and campuses are designed "to create the happiest, most productive workplace in the world". Its unorthodox workplaces and perks have been wistfully described by visiting journalists: cafés, open kitchens, sunny outdoor terraces, Lego play-spaces and gourmet cafeterias that serve free breakfast, lunch and dinner.

When Google PR staff present the company's offices, one feature is always highlighted: their state-of-the-art 'sleep pods', orb-shaped enclosures with reclining chairs and music settings to encourage sleep. Other Google offices have 'nap rooms', with airtight door locks to keep out sound and light.

Other companies have adopted similar initiatives. Nike's headquarters in Oregon has rooms where employees can sleep or meditate. The company has also rolled out flexible work start times for employees, based on their morning or evening chronotype. For the ice-cream giant Ben & Jerry's, these are not new innovations. Their headquarters has had a nap room for more than a decade.

Even New York City, whose residents take pride in the tagline 'the city that never sleeps', has seen a culture shift around sleep. A facility called Nap York opened for business in 2018 in midtown Manhattan. Referring to itself as a "wellness club", its menu of 'nap times' ranges from 15 dollars for a 30-minute power nap to 90 dollars for up to 9 hours of sleep time in a nap pod.

Nap York and similar commercial venues are cropping up as alternative means to boost energy, instead of knocking back a double espresso or reaching for a sugary treat. Seen primarily in major cities like New York and

London, such facilities hint at generally changing attitudes to daytime sleep.

The perception of sleep, and napping, has always varied across countries. Whereas Westerners have traditionally viewed daytime napping as a bit lazy, a bit slothful, this is not the case elsewhere. In Japan, for example, the very need to nap shows hard work and commitment. The Japanese office napper is a deeply conscientious worker who persists with a task until the point of exhaustion. It is termed *inemuri*, which roughly translates as 'sleeping while present'. Being present, in any form, at a tedious meeting is seen as positive. You are exhausted, but you remain, present, committed.

THE IMPORTANCE OF LIGHT

One sunny week in July, a small group of campers in their 20s and 30s headed out to the wilderness of the Rocky Mountains in Colorado. Their week was typical for backcountry campers, living in tents, away from their daily routines. Their days were spent outside in the bright sunlight, the usual mountain-desert climate. They went to bed and got up when they felt like it. They left behind their phones, tablets and laptops, and all other electronic devices were safely tucked away. In fact, they even left behind their flashlights, in an effort to return to the simplicity of the great outdoors. By the end of the week, a subtle but rather strange change had occurred. With no alarms and no set schedules, the campers had started to go to bed earlier and wake earlier, by about an hour. They were not getting more 'holiday sleep', instead their internal body clocks had shifted. In fact, 'holiday sleep' would be a misnomer – these people were no ordinary backpackers. By the end of day 7 of their camping trip, they were hustled back to the laboratory, to conclude a two-week study on light exposure and sleep timing.

Researchers at the University of Colorado, Boulder then tested the campers' levels of the hormone melatonin in their saliva every hour for 24 hours. They then compared this to the results measured before the camping week, when the "campers" had been going about their everyday lives.

The volunteers also wore light-sensing watches that collected data on light exposure, both in their normal lives and while camping. On average, they spent much of their normal life indoors, experiencing artificial light for a considerable proportion of their day. While camping, they were exposed to much brighter daytime light, then softer evening light before sunset.

Controlled by the SCN, our biological pacemaker, the hormone melatonin rises when darkness falls and drops during the day, when we are exposed to light. For this reason, it is often referred to as the 'hormone of darkness', or even the 'vampire hormone'. Melatonin also lowers body temperature, which facilitates sleep onset. After their week of camping, the volunteers' melatonin levels rose right around sunset, two hours earlier than in their everyday lives. Their internal body clocks were more closely aligned to the sun cycle. It seems that exposure to artificial light in the evening, and the tendency to experience less daylight during the day, pushed back the "natural" melatonin rise in the volunteers.

While a full week in the Rocky Mountains might not be feasible for everyone, a follow-up study by the same researchers, published in 2017, examined the effects of just one weekend of camping. This time, a small group spent two nights outdoors. Other 'control' participants stayed at home and continued as normal. After the campers got back, their melatonin level rose about 1.4 hours earlier than before. Compared to the campers, the stay-at-home group engaged in a weekend routine that will be familiar to many of us: They went to bed later and slept in longer compared to weekdays. The campers, in contrast, stuck to their weekday schedule. Having a consistent routine – going to bed and getting up at the same time every day – is a marker of good sleep.

In the summer of 2018, I spent a few weeks in the US hiking in the National Parks in Utah with some old university friends. We spent hours outside in the bright desert light, mainly walking and talking. We were not alone. In 2017, there were 4.5 million visitors to Zion National Park, known for its massive vistas of cream, pink and red sandstone cliffs. I would love to say that I slept soundly, thanks to the fresh air, the bright light, the new surroundings. Unfortunately, especially for my patient travel companions, I did not.

Most of us travel phone in hand, much of the time. My phone's camera is as powerful as any standalone camera

I've owned before, and it is convenient. In Utah, the temptation to take pictures of the scenery was constant. My good intentions of taking a break from electronic devices never actually happened. I used my smartphone with an alarming regularity across the day, and spent the evening reviewing and curating photos. Playing on my phone late into the evening probably did not help me in getting the quality sleep that I expected.

An integral part of our smartphones is that they use blue light in the screen technology. This blue light is considered to be one of the major environmental disrupters of modern sleep patterns. Blue light has been shown to affect levels of sleep-inducing melatonin more than any other wavelength of light. And light is the most powerful cue for shifting our internal body timing, our circadian clock. Our eyes have a type of receptor that detects light, not just for visual responses but for circadian rhythms. These receptors, called photosensitive retinal ganglion cells, respond to all types of light, but they are especially sensitive to blue light.

Blue light in itself is not sinister. Dawn and dusk bring changes to the blue part of the light spectrum. These natural shifts are important in setting the timing of our body clocks. But since blue light radiates from the devices we so enjoy interacting with, often in the evening, by clicking and scrolling we accumulate exposure to it. Exposure to any light source will activate the photosensitive retinal ganglion cells, but we rarely spend 20 minutes looking directly at a bright lamp. The combination of our sensitivity to blue light and prolonged device exposure is what impacts our SCN, our melatonin levels and ultimately our sleep.

Besides my smartphone habit, the other reason for my terrible holiday sleep may have been the stifling night-time heat in the desert. As the body prepares for sleep, dilating blood vessels in the skin promote heat loss. This is a key signal for falling asleep: a drop in core body temperature. But before this occurs, temperature in the distal parts of the body – the hands and feet – actually rises. We often intuitively try to speed things along with cosy socks or warm drinks, or a hot bath. These all bring blood to the surface of the skin, radiating out inner heat from the body's core.

Once the core body temperature drops enough for sleep onset, it stays lower over the night, increasing again just before we wake. Like light, temperature plays a crucial role in sleep. Lab-based studies have found that ramping up room temperature can stop the body losing heat, thereby disrupting sleep. For this reason, it is typically harder to fall asleep in a room that is too warm than in one that is too cold.

As scientists predict climate changes and more extreme weather conditions in the decades to come, this may have consequences for our sleep. Rising global temperatures may be an environmental factor, along with artificial light, that impacts future sleep quality.

OBSTACLES OLD AND NEW

ELECTRONIC DEVICES

My mother has always been a bookworm. Every night she looks forward to at least a chapter or two of a novel or, failing that, a section of the Sunday paper. Reading has been part of her pre-bedtime routine for at least thirty years. For Christmas 2017, my well-intentioned brother came up with the perfect gift for her: an iPad. This would allow her to read news and novels, with no trip to a bookstore or library. His gift was gratefully accepted – and soon had my mother swiping instead of sleeping.

Since then, several groups of scientists have tested the effects of reading, pre-bedtime, on an iPad compared to printed books. In what is now considered a landmark study, 12 young volunteers spent two weeks sleeping in a lab, where their exact bedtime routines could be controlled. For five consecutive evenings, they read digital books from iPads, and then they swapped to traditional printed books for five nights. All participants completed both reading conditions but the order they read from the iPads or printed books was shuffled. When participants read on an iPad, they took about 10 minutes longer on average to fall asleep. They also had reduced evening sleepiness, reduced melatonin secretion and less REM sleep. Even after sleeping about the same amount of time in the two reading conditions, participants were less alert in the morning after reading on an iPad.

There is much more to be read on an iPad or other tablet, but briefly summing up the biology: Tablet screens emit blue light, which impacts the SCN and suppresses melatonin's release. This prolongs wakefulness. From a psychological angle, internet-connected tablets offer diverse and stimulating content: Just as we tend to eat more food at a buffet, the Internet's cornucopia of news, social media and online shopping tempts us to stay online. This can lead to 'sleep procrastination'.

A representative survey from 2011 of 1,508 American adults found that the overwhelming majority, some 90%, used an electronic device at least a few nights per week within an hour of bedtime. A 2018 study of 815 Danish university students, with an average age of 22, monitored smartphone use over a four-week period. Most of these students used their smartphone within an hour of their self-reported bedtime. But perhaps of greater concern, 12% used their phone in the middle of the night, primarily sending text messages. About 40% had at least one night of weekday sleep interrupted by smartphone usage. More frequent smartphone usage, unsurprisingly, was associated with getting less self-reported sleep overall.

These studies indicate that we are using electronic devices at times that are incompatible with good sleep patterns. What is more, they throw up the question of cause and effect. It is often assumed that tablet use or smartphone activities, like receiving a text or call, will interrupt sleep. Conversely, however, it is plausible that the Danish students with difficulty sleeping used their phones when they were awake, to reduce boredom or as a distraction, so nightly smartphone use may be a symptom of sleep difficulties rather than a cause. Whichever direction these effects run, using electronic devices and kicking the SCN into action via light signals is not conducive to getting optimal sleep.

TAKING TECHNOLOGY TO BED

The global market for sleep aids, from mattresses to monitors, sleeping draughts and medication, was valued at USD 64.08 billion in 2021. Even so, many emerging products have little science to support claims such as 'revolutionising' bedtimes or 'curing' insomnia. Special bedding may make healthy sleepers more comfortable, but it is unlikely to reduce serious sleep difficulties.

In October 2020, the sound equipment giant Bose released the second generation of their noise-masking 'Sleepbuds II'. These earbuds are designed to minimise sleep-disrupting sounds, including snoring, traffic and voices. They also have an app that can deliver soothing soundtracks – adult lullabies if you will – to "cover and replace" noise and promote relaxation. The price of this sleep technology (250 USD) is probably equal to several years' worth of foam ear plugs from your local pharmacy.

Like other technological gear and gadgets designed to

improve sleep – including technical sleepwear, adaptive white-noise sound machines and brain-stimulating headbands – the science supporting their effects is sparse. In May 2020, there were at least 250 "white noise machine" apps available on Google Play for Android devices alone. However, a large review of the effects of continuous noise to improve sleep, in *Sleep Medicine Reviews* in 2020, reached some gloomy conclusions. The authors noted that the quality of the studies conducted so far has been "very low". They also appealed for more studies because playing continuous noise "may also negatively affect sleep and hearing".

SLEEP HYGIENE

I recently met with the Danish journalist and talk-radio host Carsten Ortmann for a broadcast discussing sleep and how to improve sleep quality. He proclaimed himself a great sleeper, proudly telling me that his bedroom doubles as an office, and all but scoffed at my first piece of advice on sleep hygiene: Keep your room for sleep and bed-related activities only.

This basic rule can help you strongly associate your bedroom with sleep. You walk into a room where virtually all you do is sleep. If you do other things in the room, like watching TV, reading or, in Carsten's case, working, you can weaken the association between the room and sleep. My response to his office-bedroom was probably thinly-veiled horror, but Carsten is convinced that his sleep is top quality. Indeed, this may well be the case, bringing us to one of the great ironies of sleep. Ask someone who is a good sleeper what they do. Most likely they will say, with some bafflement, "Nothing." People who have a relaxed attitude to sleep, who don't worry about it, who never consider whether they sleep long enough, often do. This may be similar to those who never diet but maintain a healthy weight, eating according to their appetite and rarely counting calories. Some people are simply good sleepers. Unfortunately for those who are not, sleep does not respond to effort as we might like: The harder we try to sleep, the harder it can be.

Other sleep-hygiene recommendations may sound familiar. Keep your bedroom dark, cool and quiet. Remove electronic devices. Avoid caffeine for at least 6 hours before bedtime, and alcohol too. Create a comfortable sleep environment and a wind-down routine. Such small tweaks can increase the likelihood of good-quality sleep.

SNORING AND SLEEP APNEA

In a *TIME* magazine poll from 2010 of the "Most Annoying Sounds", 'snoring' ranked alongside 'nails on a chalkboard' and 'car alarms'. And snoring is remarkably common. A 1992 study of randomly selected Danes aged between 30 and 60 years reported that around 19% of men snore habitually, far eclipsing the 8% of women who do. While snoring is not usually a sign of a serious health problem, it can be a source of intense annoyance to the snorer's partner.

Several studies have tried to quantify the consequences

of having a snoring bed partner. Thirty-seven Finnish male snorers and their partners filled in sleep diaries for two weeks. Snoring disturbed half the bed partners every night, or almost every night, and 40% of the bed partners slept in a different room at least once a week. More than a third of participants reported disharmony in their relationship, either from time to time or repeatedly, due to snoring.

In some instances, snoring can signal a more serious condition: sleep apnea. Patients with apnea experience frequent stops and starts in their breathing over the course of the night. Sleep apnea can leave the sufferer with chronic fatigue and daytime sleepiness. It can also result in a greater risk of depression, heart attacks and strokes. Of concern is that the disorder frequently goes undetected – and some scientists estimate that more than 85% of patients with sleep apnea are not diagnosed.

Sleep apnea often warrants treatment, but some patients find the cure worse than the ailment. People who do receive a diagnosis often refuse treatment, or drop out before completion. This is because the most effective treatment is not a pleasant one. Using a technique called 'continuous positive airway pressure', CPAP, air is delivered through a mask worn during the night. This can be uncomfortable and restrictive, making some wearers feel a bit like Darth Vader.

Given the discomfort of CPAP, a team of Swiss, Canadian and Dutch scientists from the University of Zurich decided to find a more palatable alternative to standard apnea treatments. They were ultimately awarded an Ig Nobel Prize in 2006 for their efforts, demonstrating that playing the didgeridoo, a hefty Australian Aboriginal wind instrument, may help alleviate sleep apnea and snoring.

Didgeridoo-playing to counteract sleep apnea was first discovered by Alex Suarez, a patient who couldn't tolerate the usual CPAP treatment. By a stroke of good fortune, he also happened to be a didgeridoo instructor. After several months of continuous practice, he noticed improvements in his own sleep. Playing the didgeridoo strengthened the muscles needed to keep the upper airways open. In a randomised clinical trial from 2006, playing a didgeridoo for 20 minutes a day, five days a week, for four months, was found to reduce daytime sleepiness and snoring. It also helped the patients' partners sleep better. According to the lead scientist, Milo Puhan of the University of Zurich, patients with sleep apnea needed to stick with their treatment regimen to keep up the benefits.

Didgeridoo-playing is unlikely to become a widespread sleep-apnea treatment – how many instructors are out there? – but it does raise an important point about treating sleep problems. Patients often find it hard to stick with their treatment plan. In the words of the former US Surgeon General, C. Everett Koop: "Drugs don't work in patients who don't take them". For any type of treatment – pharmacological or lifestyle-based – to be effective, a treatment must be practical and doable.

TRICKS, TRAINING AND THERAPY

THE PROBLEM WITH GOOD INTENTIONS

"Sleep is like a cat. It only comes to you if you ignore it."
The American novelist Gillian Flynn in her New York
Times best-selling novel "Gone Girl" drily observed the
paradox of sleep. When you truly want to rest – the night
before an exam, a performance, an important meeting –
sleep can be evasive.

People with insomnia often try really hard to sleep.
They go to bed early, they check the clock and they think
about how important it is to sleep. They often contemplate
how tired they will be in the morning if they *don't* sleep.
Meanwhile, these very thoughts, this preoccupation with
sleep, can be part of the problem.

Diverting focus away from trying to fall asleep can be a
helpful, if counter-intuitive, strategy. Termed 'paradoxical
intention therapy', this method explicitly discourages
efforts to fall asleep. At its core is the idea that trying
to control our sleep can actually disrupt it – much like
calling an uncooperative cat. To counter this, a patient is
asked to try to remain awake as long as possible. And it
is surprisingly challenging to lie in bed in a dark room,
eyes open. The instructions run something like this: "Lie

down comfortably in a darkened room and keep your eyes open. Try to keep them open 'just a little while longer'. That is your catch phrase." The paradox is that the process of trying to stay awake can make people feel sleepier. It removes some of the pressure people put on themselves to get to sleep. It actually replicates what 'good sleepers' do: fall asleep with minimal effort.

THE FORCE OF HABIT

Insomnia has often been likened to torture. In fact, sleep deprivation was a tactic favoured by the Japanese in PoW camps in World War II, and by the KGB. More recently, it has been a controversial component of the CIA's 'enhanced interrogation' techniques.

The effects of insomnia can be crippling, but there is one well-tested treatment available: Cognitive Behaviour Therapy for Insomnia, or CBT-i for short. It is recommended as the treatment of choice in many national health guidelines, above sleep medications. Usually running for 8–12 sessions, it can be delivered in person, working one-to-one with a therapist, or in a group. It is also effective as a self-help programme, accessed using a book or online.

CBT-i is comprised of a number of different elements. Some focus is on education around sleep and its importance, as well as what is termed 'sleep hygiene' – a set of behaviours that make it more likely that you will sleep well. Another element of CBT-i addresses problematic ideas, or 'cognitions', about sleep that can contribute to difficulties, such as "I need to get 8 hours of sleep" or "I've always been a bad sleeper". The most powerful component is perhaps the most counter-intuitive: sleep restriction. This is part of the 'behaviour' component of CBT-i, and it can be especially challenging for people undertaking the therapy.

It requires patients to build up their biological pressure to sleep. This is achieved by tightly restricting the window allowed for sleep, accumulating the chemical adenosine. You might set your alarm for 6 a.m. You wake at this time for a week, every day, and go to bed at 1 a.m. You get up at 6 a.m. even if you have not slept, and you do *not* nap. You also do *not* go near your bedroom until 1 a.m. This restriction resets the instinctive drive for sleep. Gradually, sleep can be extended beyond the short 5-hour window, until it begins to resemble a typical, healthy sleep pattern. Changing the sleep window in this way is typically carried out under the supervision of a healthcare professional, and involves gradual adjustments, often on a weekly basis.

Another technique, referred to as 'stimulus control', attempts to strengthen the link between being in bed and sleeping. Time lying in bed awake, or engaging in non-sleep activities like streaming videos, reading or eating, is discouraged. Patients are instructed to get out of bed if they are not asleep within a given period, say 20 minutes. Over time, being in bed comes to be strongly associated with sleep.

CBT-i now has a large body of trials demonstrating its efficacy. Long-term studies of patients show that people continue to sleep better even after treatment ends. Following CBT-i takes effort and commitment – like didgeridoo playing – with the key techniques requiring practice, lifestyle changes and considerable discomfort. It is not surprising that on average about 17% of patients drop out of CBT-i, but those who do finish the treatment tend to benefit.

SLEEPING PILLS

About 4% of all American adults over the age of 20 used prescription medication in the prior month, according to a 2013 report from the Centers for Disease Control and Prevention. Even greater numbers take over-the-counter sleep medications.

In 1993, the sleep medication market experienced a major shift, when the French company Sanofi introduced a drug called zolpidem, brand-named 'Ambien'. Classed as a hypnotic drug, it quickly dominated sleep-medication prescriptions, making the company more than 1 billion US dollars in annual sales. For a period, this drug enjoyed a near-monopoly, which rarely occurs in the world of prescription medications.

After one of the Kennedy family blamed a 2006 car accident on disorientation from Ambien, the potential unwanted effects of the drug began to receive widespread attention. Now, its prescriptions must include strong warnings about side effects such as sleep-eating, sleep-walking and sleep-driving.

Furthermore, when people stop taking zolpidem, or

other medications, their sleep often reverts to its previous state. This can create a cycle of dependency, which, along with concerns about side effects, means that medications are only really recommended in the short term. Healthcare guidelines in many countries also advise that such medications are prescribed only after behaviour therapy and other non-pharmacological options have been tried first.

MELATONIN: THE 'NATURAL' OPTION

Deep in the brain, the pineal gland, controlled by the SCN, increases production of melatonin in the evening, as light fades. This encourages sleep, and melatonin production ramps down in the early morning hours. Synthetic forms of this hormone are also sold in many European countries and in the US as an over-the-counter dietary supplement. Because melatonin is found in common foods, including nuts, seeds and olive oil, it is classed as a nutritional supplement rather than a drug in many to numerous countries.

An analysis carried out in 2013, pooling the results of 19 clinical trials, has given us a reasonable picture of the impact of melatonin on adults with a diagnosed sleep disorder. Patients who were given melatonin tablets fell asleep on average 7 minutes faster than those given placebo tablets. They also slept a total of 8 minutes longer than the placebo group. These are modest effects, but they are still considered relevant by doctors because melatonin has fewer side effects than other medications.

In contrast to caffeine, melatonin has a short half-life of around an hour. This means that melatonin's major effect should be in shortening the time it takes to fall asleep. Because it does not linger in the body, it is not expected to reduce night time awakenings, or improve the overall quality of sleep.

Melatonin and numerous other drugs have been tested on patients with insomnia, and there is evidence that they work, to varying degrees. However, when the American Academy of Sleep Medicine reviewed this evidence in 2017, with the aim of providing clinicians with guidelines, they expressed deep concern. They noted that the quality and availability of evidence for many approved sleep drugs was "sorely limited". For all 14 recommendations made by the Academy, evidence was graded as "weak". This means doctors must use their clinical judgement and experience when prescribing sleep medications, in the absence of a body of high-quality studies.

TO TRACK OR NOT TO TRACK

Prince Harry of the UK was spotted wearing an Oura Ring while on holiday in October 2018 with his new wife, the American actress Megan Markle. This is not the expected jewellery choice for a UK royal, but it hints at how mainstream sleep trackers have become. The ring tracks body temperature and blood-volume pulse and uses sensors, including an accelerometer and a gyroscope, to track body movements.

Oura claims to use physiological signals – a

combination of motion, heart rate, heart-rate variability and pulse-wave variability amplitude – along with machine learning to calculate sleep and wake time and various sleep stages. It has been described as a "tiny Fitbit for your finger", although the makers of the Oura would likely balk at the comparison with the more accessible and less expensive Fibit.

The Fitbit is one of a plethora of wearable wrist devices now available. It is quite likely that you have a wearable device yourself, or know someone who does, to track sleep and activity. Most smartwatches from the major device manufacturers also include sleep tracking as a standard feature. They typically use wrist movements, or lack of them, to determine whether the wearer has fallen asleep. The newer generations of trackers include measurements of blood flow, and integrate these into their sleep estimate. Unfortunately for academic researchers, these commercial devices use proprietary algorithms to calculate sleep, so we do not know exactly how they arrive at their estimations.

Compared to the 'gold standard' of sleep measurement – laboratory-based polysomnography – commercial trackers tend to overestimate total sleep time. This is unsurprising: Being very still and not moving your wrist does *not* equate to being asleep.

In fact, in one of my own studies from 2018, we asked volunteers to wear Fitbits for 8 weeks. They were quite irritated by the device's inaccuracy. For example, one volunteer complained that periods of reading in bed in the morning were recorded as sleep. Other volunteers found the watch so annoying to wear that they took it off after a few nights. Yet others enjoyed the tracking experience so much that they bought their own devices at the end of the study.

Commercial wearable trackers, especially newer models, provide a reasonable but not entirely precise estimate of sleep opportunity. This information may be helpful for setting sleep routines and tracking bedtime regularity. Simply knowing what your sleep patterns are may allow you to adjust your schedule to ensure an adequate sleep window of 7–9 hours. At least that's the idea.

The act of tracking does not necessarily lead to more sleep. Unlike exercise or drinking extra water, conscientiously striving to get more sleep can, in fact, be counter-productive, especially if it leads to anxious, negative thoughts around sleep. Such thoughts can provoke a vicious circle of arousal, an inability to relax enough to sleep and then further anxiety about the detrimental effects of poor sleep.

Like every new technology, there are potential downsides to sleep trackers and reasons for cautious uptake. For many people, however, if sleep tracking is light-hearted and does not heighten worry, it may be a useful catalyst for constructive behaviour change. As an old adage in medicine says, "What's measured is managed."

There is no downside to making sure you consistently get a good night's sleep. If you disrupt sleep, you disrupt attention, food intake and physical co-ordination. On the upside, if you can improve your sleep, there is a potential for improving your well-being across many domains.

Short periods of sleep deprivation are not the end of the world. Just as one bad meal won't cause significant weight gain, one bad night won't significantly disrupt your health. There may be some short-term unpleasant consequences, but your body will return to its normal state fairly quickly. For sleep loss, you may well feel lousy the next day too, but the effects of a poor night's sleep, like those of eating a bit of junk food, will soon dissipate.

The problem arises when we systematically and consistently undervalue sleep. This may, in part, be down to the lack of a clear, simple explanation for why we sleep. It is hard to prioritise a behaviour when we don't understand its exact function. But scientists agree: An over-tired brain is not at its best.

Many of us are sleep procrastinators. There are so many things in the waking world that seem more exciting, more pressing. But to quote the celebrated diaries of the seventeenth-century English writer Samuel Pepys: "And So to Bed".